EmpowerHer Essence

A 15-Day Journey to Rediscover and Celebrate Your Feminine Wellness"

This Book Belongs To:

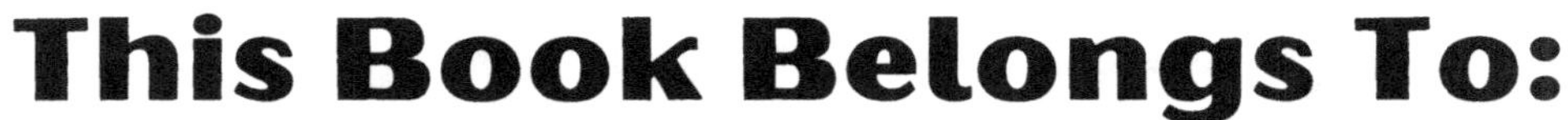

Welcome, beautiful soul, to "EmpowerHer Essence: A 15-Day Journey to Rediscover and Celebrate Your Feminine Wellness." This is not just a book, but a sacred journey to deepen your connection with the most intimate and powerful part of yourself - your yoni.

The term 'yoni', rooted in ancient Sanskrit, transcends the biological definition of the female reproductive system. It represents the divine feminine, the source of all creation, and the seat of intuition and life force. In a world that often distances us from our bodies, this journal seeks to bridge that gap, encouraging you to embrace, understand, and nourish your yoni.

Throughout the next 15 days, you will be guided through reflections, activities, and affirmations that aim to foster a profound sense of love, respect, and understanding for your yoni. Each day is an invitation to look inward, to listen, and to celebrate the wisdom your body holds. Whether you're on a path of healing, or discovery, or simply wishing to cultivate a deeper relationship with your feminine essence, this journal is here to support and uplift you.

Before you begin, remember:

- There's no right or wrong way to feel. Every woman's journey with her yoni is unique. Honor your feelings and experiences, knowing they are valid

- Trust the process. Some days might feel challenging, while others might bring joy and clarity. Embrace each day as a step closer to your inner truth.

- This is a safe space. Let this journal be your sanctuary. A place of non-judgment, where you can be honest, raw, and open.

As you turn the pages, know that with each word and stroke of your pen, you are weaving a deeper connection with your yoni and, ultimately, with yourself. Let's embark on this sacred journey together, uncovering the mysteries and wonders of our feminine essence.

With love and light...

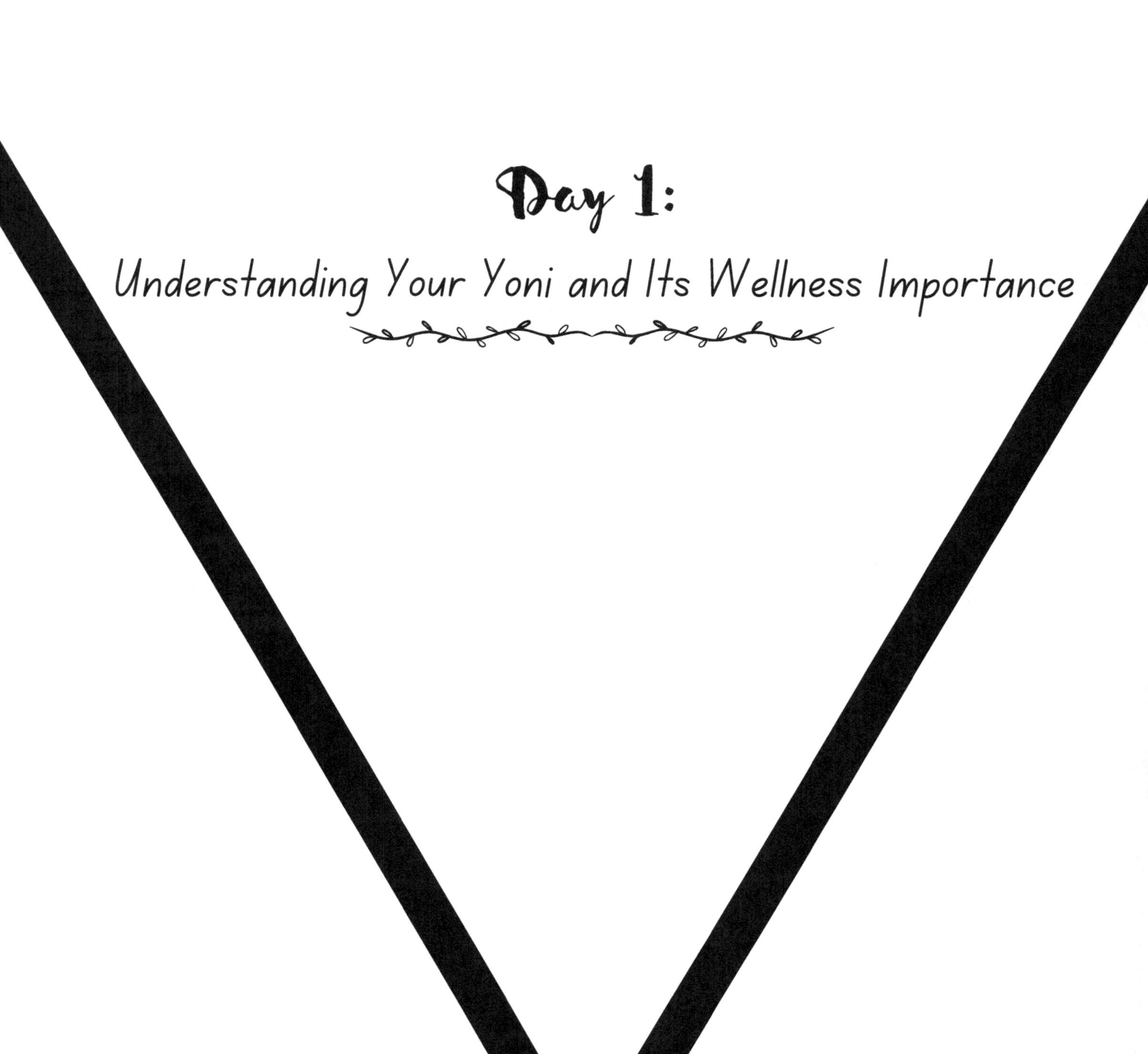

Day 1:

Understanding Your Yoni and Its Wellness Importance

Day 1:

Understanding Your Yoni and Its Wellness Importance

Description of the Yoni:

The term "yoni" originates from Sanskrit and is often used to refer to the female reproductive system, encompassing the vagina, uterus, and ovaries. However, beyond its anatomical definition, the yoni represents so much more. In many cultures and spiritual practices, it's regarded as a sacred space, symbolizing the source of life, creativity, and feminine energy. The yoni is not just a physical entity but also an embodiment of a woman's essence, power, and connection to the universe.

Importance of Yoni Wellness:

Yoni wellness is paramount not just for reproductive health but also for emotional, mental, and spiritual well-being. Here's why:

Physical Health: Like any other part of the body, the yoni is susceptible to imbalances, infections, and diseases. Regular attention and care can prevent many common ailments and ensure that any concerns are addressed early.

Emotional Connection: How one feels about their yoni can deeply impact their self-esteem, body image, and emotional well-being. Embracing and loving the yoni can foster a profound sense of self-love and acceptance.

Sexual Well-being: A healthy yoni plays a significant role in sexual pleasure, comfort, and intimacy. By understanding and caring for the yoni, one can enhance their sexual experiences and cultivate deeper connections with partners.

Spiritual Significance: For many, the yoni is a gateway to the divine feminine, a source of creative energy, and a connection to Mother Earth. By nurturing yoni wellness, one can also tap into this reservoir of spiritual energy.

Holistic Health: The yoni is interconnected with other systems in the body. Its health can influence hormonal balance, urinary function, and overall pelvic health. Thus, yoni wellness is integral to holistic health.

Reflection

Having read about the significance and role of the yoni in your life, how do you currently relate to yours? Are there areas you feel you've neglected or want to explore further?

____

____

____

____

____

____

____

____

Todays Affirmation:

"My yoni is a sacred space of power and creativity."

"I am in tune with the unique rhythms of my body."

"Every part of me deserves love and acceptance, including my yoni."

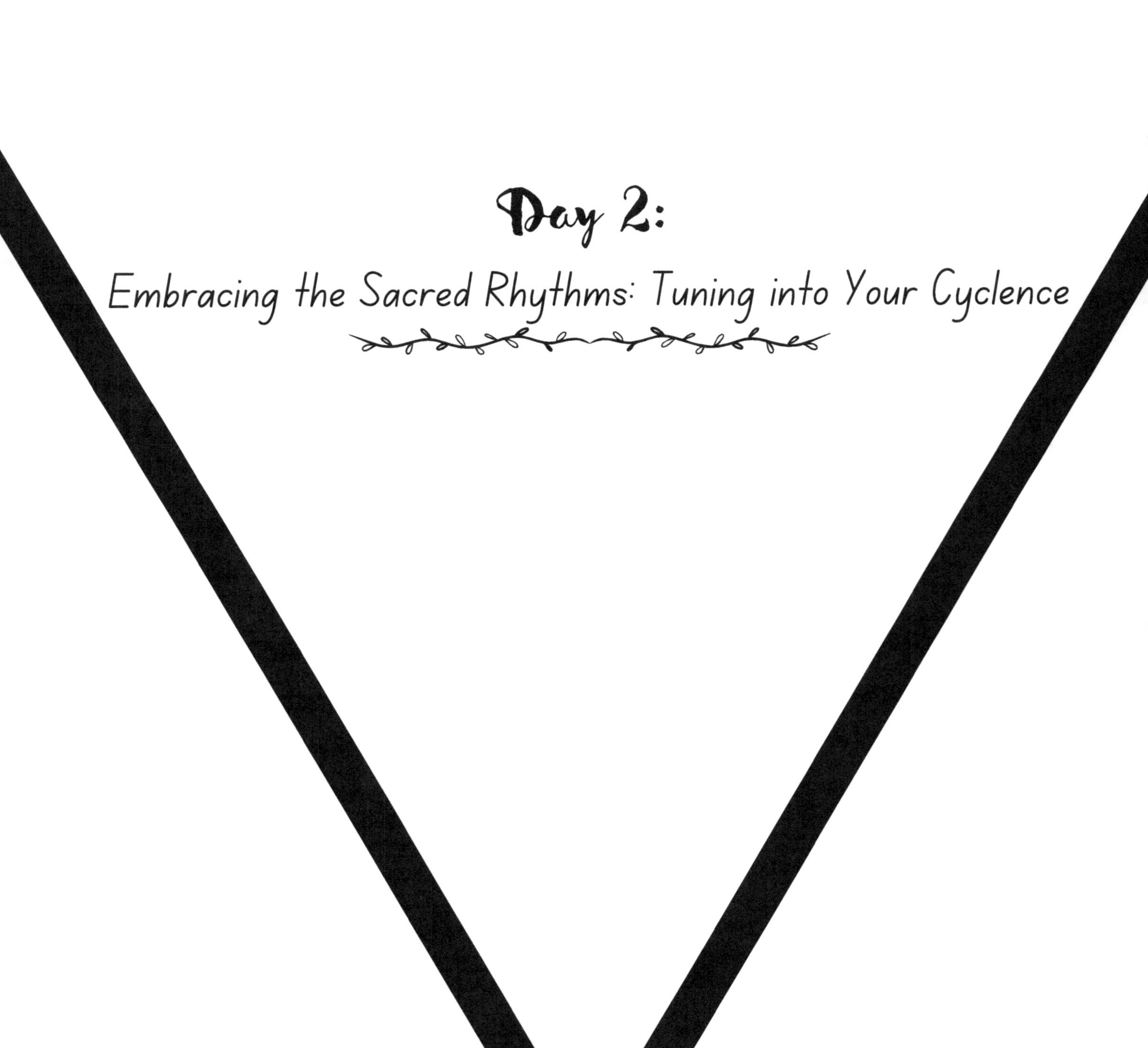
Day 2:

Embracing the Sacred Rhythms: Tuning into Your Cyclence

Day 2:

Embracing the Sacred Rhythms: Tuning into Your Cyclence

Our bodies, especially our yonis, operate in rhythms and cycles, much like nature itself. The moon's waxing and waning mirror the ebb and flow of our menstrual cycles. Today, we'll delve into understanding and embracing these sacred rhythms, recognizing the beauty and power of our menstrual cycle.

Activity:

Menstrual Cycle Mapping: Draw a circle on the next page and divide it into four equal parts, representing the four phases of your menstrual cycle: menstrual, follicular, ovulatory, and luteal.

Menstrual Phase: When you menstruate. A time for rest, reflection, and renewal.

- *Follicular Phase:* After menstruating, leading up to ovulation. A period of growth, energy, and creativity.

- *Ovulatory Phase:* When you're most fertile. A time for communication, connection, and expression.

- *Luteal Phase:* After ovulation, leading up to menstruation. A period for slowing down, self-care, and introspection.

Reflect on each phase and jot down how you generally feel emotionally, physically, and mentally during each one. If you don't menstruate or have irregular cycles, reflect on your natural rhythms and what you notice throughout a typical month.

Menstrual Cycle Mapping:

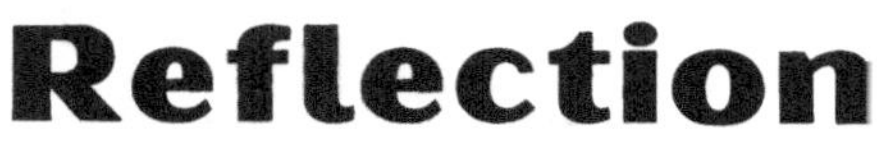

Reflection

1. How aware are you of the different phases of your menstrual cycle? Do you notice shifts in your energy, mood, or desires?
2. Have you ever felt pressured to remain consistent in your energy and mood, despite the natural fluctuations of your cycle?
3. How can you honor and care for yourself better during each phase?

____

____

____

____

____

____

____

Todays Affirmation:

"I am in harmony with the natural rhythms of my body.
Each phase of my cycle brings its unique gifts and
lessons."

"My yoni is a source of wisdom, strength, and vitality."

"I embrace the journey of connecting deeply with my feminine essence."

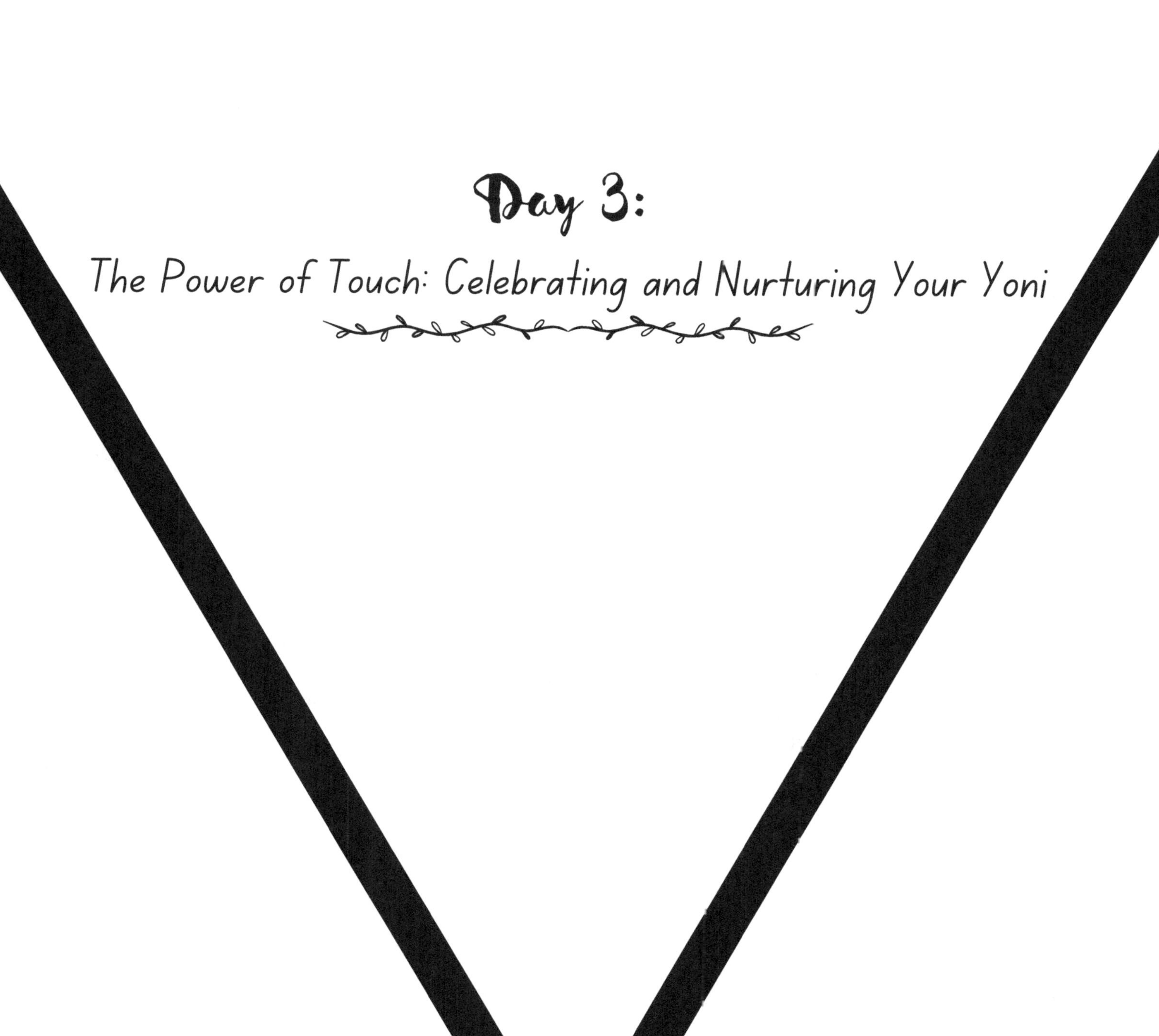

Day 3:

The Power of Touch: Celebrating and Nurturing Your Yoni

Day 3:

The Power of Touch: Celebrating and Nurturing Your Yoni

Touch is one of the most fundamental forms of connection and healing. Just as we apply touch to comfort a pain or soothe an ache elsewhere in our body, our yoni too can benefit immensely from gentle, mindful touch. Today, we focus on understanding the importance of touch in nurturing our yoni and integrating simple, non-sexual self-care practices that fortify our connection to this sacred space.

Self-Care Tips:

Warmth: A warm compress or a heat pad can be a wonderful way to soothe menstrual cramps or simply to relax the pelvic area. Warmth encourages blood flow and can be deeply comforting.

Breath Work: Focusing your breath on the pelvic region can have a calming and grounding effect. Deep, intentional breaths can help release tension and create a sense of connection.

Gentle Massage: Using a natural oil like coconut or almond, give yourself a gentle lower abdomen massage in circular motions. This can be great for reducing bloating, easing discomfort, or simply promoting relaxation.

Hydration: Drinking adequate water supports overall well-being, but it also ensures that the yoni remains healthy, aiding in natural lubrication and toxin removal.

Yoni Steams (with caution): This ancient practice involves sitting over a pot of herbal-infused steam, which is believed to cleanse and rejuvenate. If you're interested, research herbs that resonate with you and consult with a professional before trying. Note: Avoid during menstruation or if you're pregnant.

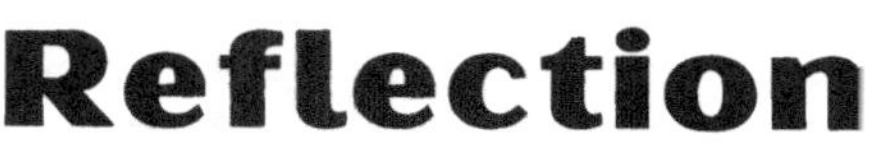

Reflection

1. How often do you consciously attend to your yoni outside of hygiene routines?
2. Were there any self-care practices mentioned above that resonated with you or that you'd like to try?
3. How did the Yoni breathing exercise feel? Did you notice any areas of tension or release?

Todays Affirmation:

"My yoni is deserving of care, attention, and gentle touch.
Through nurturing practices, I strengthen my connection to my
sacred feminine essence."

"With each act of self-care, I honor and cherish the sacred temple
that is my yoni."

"In nurturing my yoni, I embrace the fullness of my feminine power and wisdom."

Day 4:

Yoni's Ecosystem: Understanding and Balancing Your Vaginal Flora

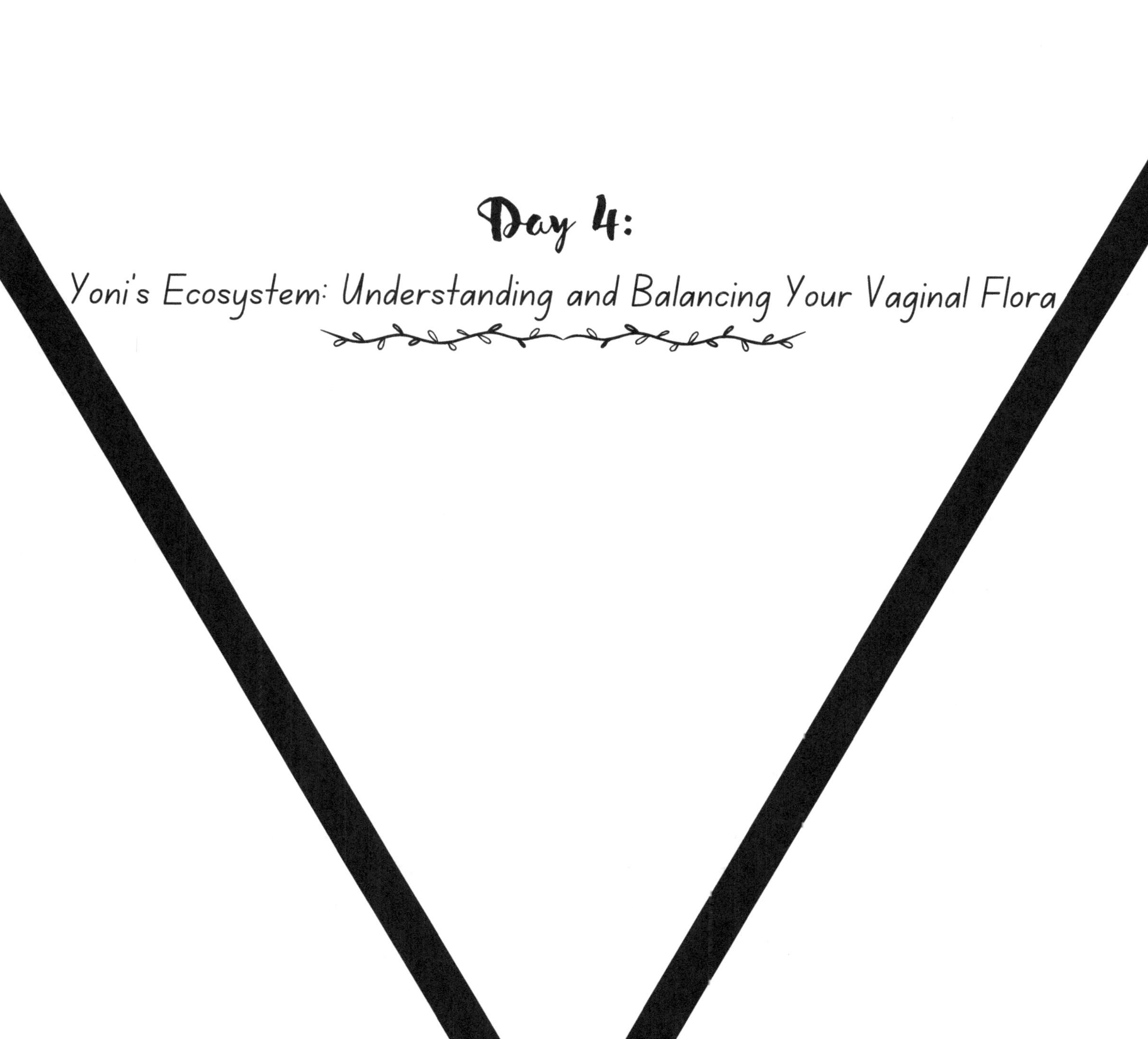

Day 4:

Yoni's Ecosystem: Understanding and Balancing Your Vaginal Flora

Much like the delicate balance of an ecosystem in nature, our yoni too has its own intricate ecosystem. It's home to a variety of microorganisms, primarily beneficial bacteria, which play an essential role in maintaining its health and preventing infections. Today, we'll dive into understanding this unique ecosystem and how we can support its optimal balance.

Understanding the Vaginal Flora:

The vaginal environment is acidic, maintained by the predominant bacteria called lactobacilli. These beneficial bacteria produce lactic acid, keeping the pH low (acidic) and preventing harmful pathogens from thriving. Disruptions to this balance can lead to conditions like bacterial vaginosis or yeast infections.

Activities and Practices:

Yoni pH Test:

- *Purpose:* To be aware of the pH balance of your yoni.
- *How-to:* Purchase a vaginal pH test kit from a pharmacy. Use it as per instructions, typically best done outside of your menstrual period. Healthy vaginal pH is usually between 3.8 to 4.5. If you find consistent deviations, consider seeing a healthcare professional.

Dietary Journaling:

- *Purpose:* Food plays a significant role in our overall health, including the health of our yoni.
- *How-to:* For a week, maintain a journal of your daily food intake. At the end of the week, reflect on how often you consumed fermented foods (like yogurt, kimchi, or sauerkraut) which can support beneficial bacteria. (A food journal has been made available to you, page 21)

Self-Care Tips for a Balanced Vaginal Flora:

Favor Cotton Underwear: Cotton is breathable and can help prevent the build-up of moisture, reducing the chance of bacterial overgrowth.

Avoid Douching: The vagina is self-cleaning, and douching can disrupt the natural balance of bacteria. Instead, wash with just warm water or a mild, unscented soap if necessary.

Stay Hydrated: Drinking ample water supports overall health and ensures efficient flushing out of toxins.

Eat Probiotic-Rich Foods: Foods like yogurt, kefir, kombucha, and other fermented items can help replenish and support beneficial bacteria.

Change Menstrual Products Regularly: Whether you use pads, tampons, or menstrual cups, ensure they're changed/cleaned regularly to prevent bacterial overgrowth.

Embrace Day 4 as an opportunity to deepen your understanding of the intricate workings of your yoni. Recognizing and respecting its delicate balance empowers you to make informed choices for your well-being.

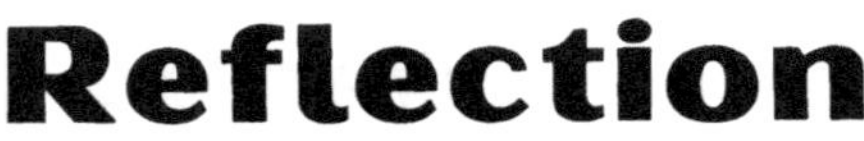

Reflection

1. Were you aware of the importance of pH balance in your yoni's health?
2. How often do you incorporate probiotic-rich foods in your diet?
3. Are there any habits you might consider changing to better support your vaginal flora?

____

____

____

____

____

____

____

____

Todays Affirmation:

"In nurturing the delicate balance of my yoni, I foster its strength, health, and vitality."

"Every choice I make echoes my commitment to the harmonious ecosystem within me."

"I honor the natural balance of my yoni and support its flourishing ecosystem. My body's wisdom guides me in maintaining harmony."

FOOD JOURNAL

WEEK: _______________

Breakfast ____________________

Lunch ____________________

Dinner ____________________

Snacks ____________________

Bottles of water ○ ○ ○ ○ ○

Breakfast ____________________

Lunch ____________________

Dinner ____________________

Snacks ____________________

Bottles of water ○ ○ ○ ○ ○

Breakfast ____________________

Lunch ____________________

Dinner ____________________

Snacks ____________________

Bottles of water ○ ○ ○ ○ ○

Breakfast ____________________

Lunch ____________________

Dinner ____________________

Snacks ____________________

Bottles of water ○ ○ ○ ○ ○

Breakfast ____________________

Lunch ____________________

Dinner ____________________

Snacks ____________________

Bottles of water ○ ○ ○ ○ ○

Breakfast ____________________

Lunch ____________________

Dinner ____________________

Snacks ____________________

Bottles of water ○ ○ ○ ○ ○

Breakfast ____________________

Lunch ____________________

Dinner ____________________

Snacks ____________________

Bottles of water ○ ○ ○ ○ ○

NOTES:

____

____

____

____

____

Day 5:

Inner Wisdom: Decoding the Messages of Your Yoni

Day 5:

Inner Wisdom: Decoding the Messages of Your Yoni

Our bodies are constantly communicating with us, sending signals about our well-being, needs, and imbalances. The yoni, as a powerful center of intuition and sensation, has its own set of messages. Today, we explore the art of tuning in, understanding, and honoring the whispers and signals of the yoni, guiding us towards holistic wellness.

Activities:

Sensation Mapping:

Purpose: To become more aware of the physical sensations in your yoni.

How-to: Sit comfortably and close your eyes. Take deep breaths, directing your focus to your yoni. Without touching, simply notice any sensations – warmth, tingling, tension, relaxation, etc. Journal any feelings or sensations you detect.

Intuitive Journaling:

Purpose: To decode the deeper, intuitive messages your yoni might be conveying.

How-to: In a quiet space, ask your yoni if it has any messages for you – about your health, relationships, boundaries, or desires. Write down any impressions, feelings, or thoughts that arise, even if they seem unrelated or random.

Self-Care Tips for Tuning into Your Yoni's Messages:

- Mindful Breathing: Spending just a few minutes each day focusing on deep, abdominal breathing can help you center yourself and tune in to your body's signals.

- Regular Check-ins: Set aside a specific time daily, perhaps before bedtime or during morning rituals, to mentally check in with your yoni. Ask: How do you feel today?

- Warm Baths: A warm bath, especially with calming essential oils like lavender or chamomile, can be both relaxing and a chance to connect with your yoni.

- Limit Irritants: Be mindful of products used near or in the yoni. Avoiding scented soaps, lotions, or washes can reduce the chance of irritation and help you more clearly discern any messages or sensations.

- Stay Hydrated: Water supports overall body health, ensuring efficient communication between different body systems.

-

Todays Affirmation:

"In nurturing the delicate balance of my yoni, I foster its strength, health, and vitality."

"Every choice I make echoes my commitment to the harmonious ecosystem within me."

"I honor the natural balance of my yoni and support its flourishing ecosystem. My body's wisdom guides me in maintaining harmony."

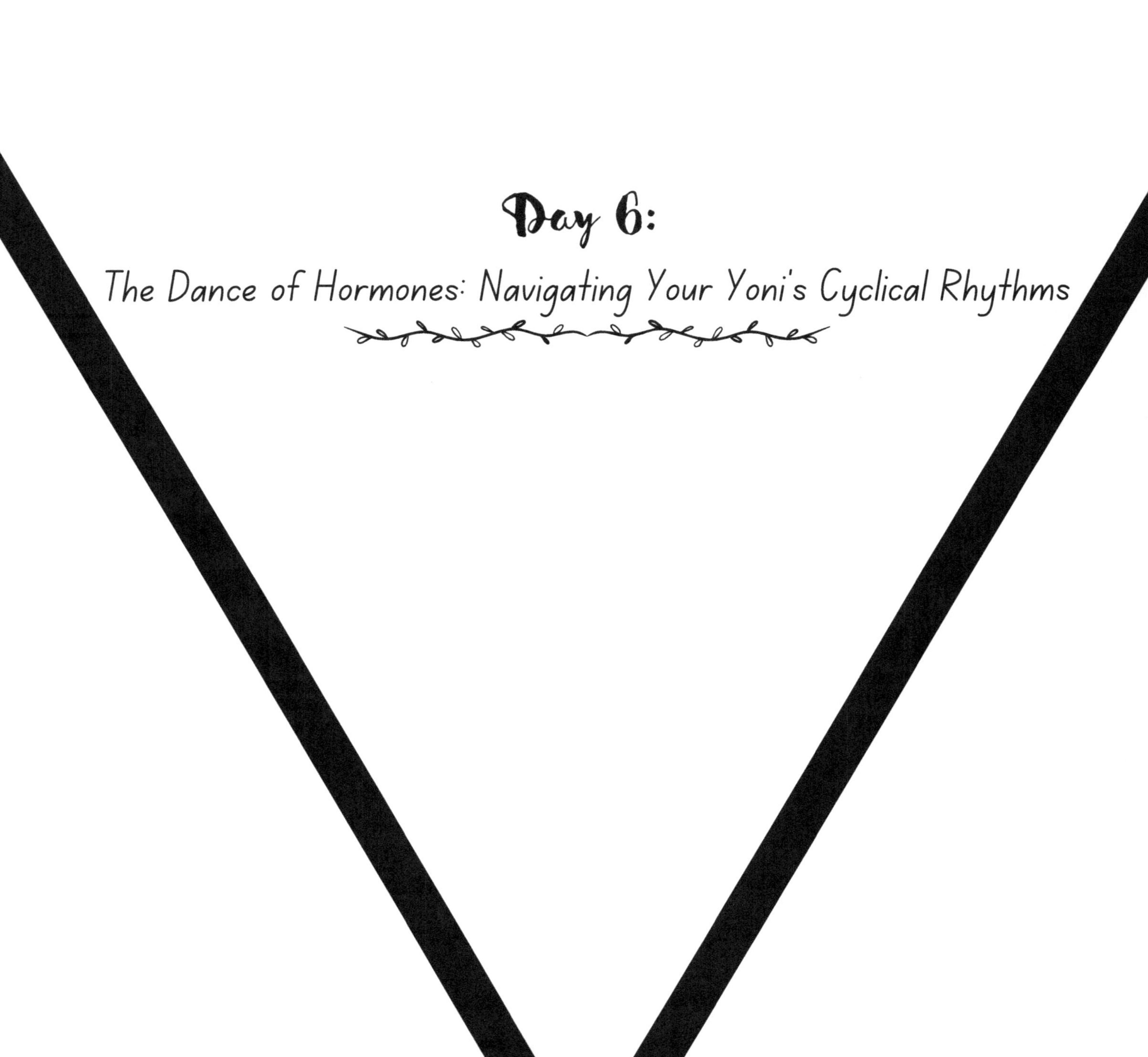

Day 6:

The Dance of Hormones: Navigating Your Yoni's Cyclical Rhythms

Day 6:

The Dance of Hormones: Navigating Your Yoni's Cyclical Rhythms

Understanding the natural rhythms of our body is essential for every woman. The hormonal changes that occur during the menstrual cycle affect not only the cycle itself but also our mood, energy levels, and overall well-being. In this journey, we explore this beautiful ballet of hormones that ebb and flow throughout the month.

The Hormonal Ballet:

Throughout a typical menstrual cycle, hormone levels fluctuate. Two main hormones, estrogen, and progesterone, play pivotal roles.

Follicular Phase (Days 1-14): Beginning with the first day of menstruation and ending with ovulation. Estrogen levels rise, leading to increased energy, mood elevation, and optimism.

Luteal Phase (Days 15-28): After ovulation, progesterone levels rise, sometimes leading to mood swings, fatigue, or PMS symptoms in some women.

Understanding these changes can help you plan activities, self-care routines, and even important decisions around your cycle, harnessing your body's natural strengths at various times.

Activities:

Cycle Tracking:

- ***Purpose:*** To become attuned to your body's hormonal rhythms.
- ***How-to:*** Use a journal or app to mark the start and end of your menstrual period, noting any significant mood or energy shifts, cravings, or physical sensations.

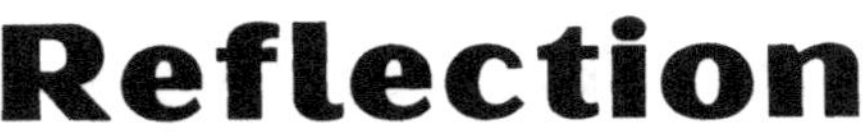

1. Were you previously aware of the two main phases of your menstrual cycle?
2. Have you noticed specific patterns or feelings associated with each phase?
3. How can you adjust your daily routines or activities to align better with your hormonal rhythms?

Todays Affirmation:

"I embrace the innate rhythms of my body, flowing in harmony with my hormones.

"In the ebb and flow of my hormones, I find the strength and wisdom of my femininity."

"Every phase of my cycle holds its own magic, and I honor each with grace and understanding."

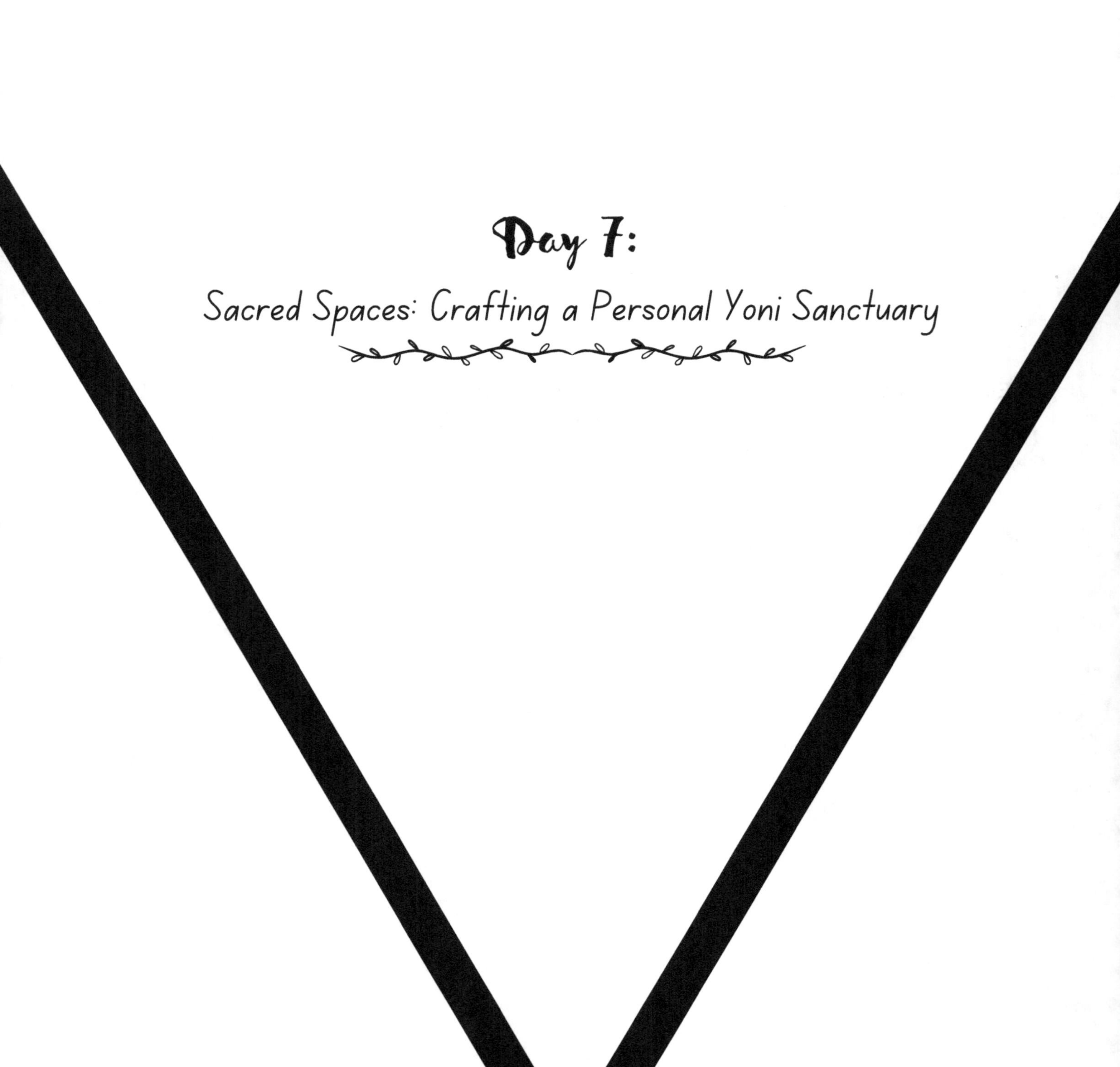

Day 7:

Sacred Spaces: Crafting a Personal Yoni Sanctuary

Day 7:

Sacred Spaces: Crafting a Personal Yoni Sanctuary

Our surroundings have a powerful impact on our overall health and happiness. In this discussion, we'll explore the creation of a sanctuary - a space solely dedicated to yoni wellness and self-reflection. This personal haven will serve as a grounding point where you can consistently reconnect with your yoni, ensuring its proper care and understanding.

The Essence of a Sanctuary:

A sanctuary is more than just a physical space. It embodies safety, peace, and healing energy. While the specifics can vary greatly depending on individual preferences, the intent remains the same: a sacred place to honor and nourish your yoni.

Self-Practices:

Sanctuary Setup:

- *Purpose:* To establish a dedicated space for yoni practices and reflections.
- *How-to:* Choose a quiet corner in your home, perhaps in your bedroom or a separate room if available. Adorn it with items that make you feel connected and serene, such as crystals, candles, incense, or yoni-inspired art.

Daily Moments of Gratitude:

- *Purpose:* To foster appreciation for your yoni and its innate wisdom.
- *How-to:* In your sanctuary, spend a few minutes each day expressing gratitude for your yoni. Journal or verbalize the things you appreciate about it – its strength, resilience, wisdom, and its role in experiences or pleasures.

Exercises:

1. **Yoni Visualization:**
   - **Purpose:** Enhance connection and awareness.
   - **How-to:** Sit comfortably in your sanctuary. Close your eyes and breathe deeply. Visualize your yoni as a source of light, warmth, and energy. Imagine this light expanding, filling your entire body with its glow, and grounding you.
2. **Breath Awareness Practice:**
   - **Purpose:** Foster deeper connection between breath and yoni.
   - **How-to:** In a seated or lying position, place one hand on your chest and the other on your lower abdomen. Inhale deeply, feeling your abdomen rise, drawing energy towards your yoni. Exhale, visualizing any tension or negativity releasing.

Self-Care Tips:

Regular Cleansing: Ensure your sanctuary remains a place of positive energy by routinely clearing it. You can smudge with sage, sprinkle saltwater, or simply open windows to let fresh air cleanse the space.

Personal Touch: Add personal items that resonate with you – perhaps a favorite blanket, cushion, or even a yoni egg if you use one.

Nature Connection: Incorporate elements of nature, such as plants or flowing water, to enhance the grounding and healing properties of your sanctuary.

<u>Natural Soothing Rinse</u>

Creating and using a natural feminine cleanse can be a ritual of self-care, but it's vital to approach it with knowledge and awareness. Your yoni is a delicate ecosystem, and its well-being is paramount.

Ingredients:
1. Warm purified water: Acts as a gentle base for the cleanse.
2. A tablespoon of organic apple cider vinegar (with the 'mother'): Helps maintain a healthy pH balance. Apple cider vinegar has natural acidic properties that can balance the yoni's pH, which is slightly acidic.
3. 1-2 drops of lavender essential oil: Known for its calming and anti-inflammatory properties. It can also be beneficial for its mild antiseptic qualities.
4. 1-2 drops of chamomile essential oil: Chamomile can be soothing and anti-inflammatory.

Directions:
1. Start by ensuring that your hands and all tools or containers used are clean.
2. Take a bowl of warm purified water (about a quart or liter). Ensure the water is not too hot.
3. Add the tablespoon of organic apple cider vinegar to the water.
4. Add the drops of lavender and chamomile essential oil.
5. Stir gently to mix the ingredients.

Usage:
1. After a shower or bath, pour the mixture into a clean squeeze bottle or a feminine hygiene douche bag.
2. With clean hands, gently cleanse the external parts of the yoni. Avoid douching or pushing the mixture internally, as this can disrupt the natural flora inside.
3. Pat dry with a clean, soft towel.

Notes:

- Always use this cleanse externally. Douching or introducing any liquid internally can disrupt the natural balance of beneficial bacteria in the vagina.
- If you experience any irritation or unusual symptoms, discontinue use and consult a healthcare professional.
- Remember that our bodies are unique, so what works for one person might not work for another. Always pay attention to how your body responds.

Todays Affirmation:

"In the sacred space I've created, I honor the divine wisdom and power of my yoni."

"My sanctuary mirrors the beauty and strength of my inner essence, grounding me in love and self-awareness."

"In my sanctuary, I find solace and strength. Here, I honor and celebrate the divine essence of my yoni."

Day 8:

Embracing the Seasons: Celebrating the Stages of Yoni Life

Day 8:

Embracing the Seasons: Celebrating the Stages of Yoni Life

The yoni, just like nature, goes through seasons throughout a woman's life. These seasons represent the different stages of womanhood - from menstruation to menopause and beyond. Each stage brings its own lessons, challenges, and celebrations. Today, we will explore and gain deeper insights into these stages, appreciating the beauty and significance of each one.

The Seasons of the Yoni:

Blossoming (Menarche):

Physiological Changes: This is when a young girl has her first menstrual cycle. Hormones like estrogen and progesterone begin to surge, leading to the development of secondary sexual characteristics such as breast growth, widening of the hips, and the beginning of menstrual cycles.

Emotional Journey: This stage often comes with a whirlwind of emotions due to hormonal changes. There's excitement about entering womanhood, but also apprehension about the changes. Societal and cultural beliefs around menstruation can impact self-perception and confidence.

Celebration & Connection: Embrace this phase by ensuring there's open communication about menstrual health, body changes, and emotional well-being. Encouraging a ritual or ceremony can also validate and honor this rite of passage.

Fertility and Reproduction:

Physiological Changes: Women in this phase experience regular menstrual cycles. The body prepares for potential pregnancy every month, and there's an ebb and flow of hormones associated with the menstrual cycle phases.

Emotional Journey: This season is often marked by exploration — whether that's in relationships, career, or self-identity. For some, there might be the desire for motherhood, while for others, it might be a time of deep personal growth and discovery.

Celebration & Connection: It's essential to remain connected with one's body, recognizing and celebrating fertility signs, and making informed decisions about reproductive health.

Empowerment (Midlife and Pre-Menopause):

Physiological Changes: Hormonal levels, especially estrogen, start to decline. Women might notice changes in their menstrual cycle patterns, and symptoms like hot flashes or mood fluctuations might begin.

Emotional Journey: There's often a reevaluation of personal goals, desires, and life trajectory. Many women feel empowered by their accumulated life experiences, while others might grapple with the idea of aging and the changes it brings.

Celebration & Connection: This is a time for reflection and asserting one's needs. Engaging in self-care, seeking support groups, or therapy can be beneficial.

Wisdom (Menopause and Post-Menopause):

Physiological Changes: Menstrual cycles cease entirely, and there's a marked decrease in hormones like estrogen. This change can affect bone density, skin health, and even heart health.

Emotional Journey: There's a profound sense of transition. While some women embrace the freedom from menstrual cycles, others might mourn the end of their reproductive years. There's also a deep well of wisdom and experiences that come to the forefront.

Celebration & Connection: It's vital to prioritize health, focusing on bone health, cardiovascular wellness, and emotional well-being. Joining support groups, engaging in community activities, or taking up new hobbies can be rejuvenating.

Self-Care Tips for Each Season:

- *Blossoming:* Educate yourself about menstrual health, using natural and organic menstrual products.

- *Fertility and Reproduction:* Engage in regular check-ups, practice safe intimacy, and nurture your emotional well-being.

- *Empowerment:* Consider practices like yoga or meditation to navigate hormonal shifts and emotional changes gracefully.

- *Wisdom:* Ensure bone health through diet and exercise, engage in brain-stimulating activities, and prioritize emotional well-being.

Todays Affirmation:

"Each phase of my yoni's evolution is a testament to my resilience, strength, and the beauty of womanhood."

"With every season of my yoni's journey, I deepen my connection to the rhythms of life and nature."

"Every season of my yoni's journey is a dance of transformation, and I embrace each stage with grace, understanding, and celebration."

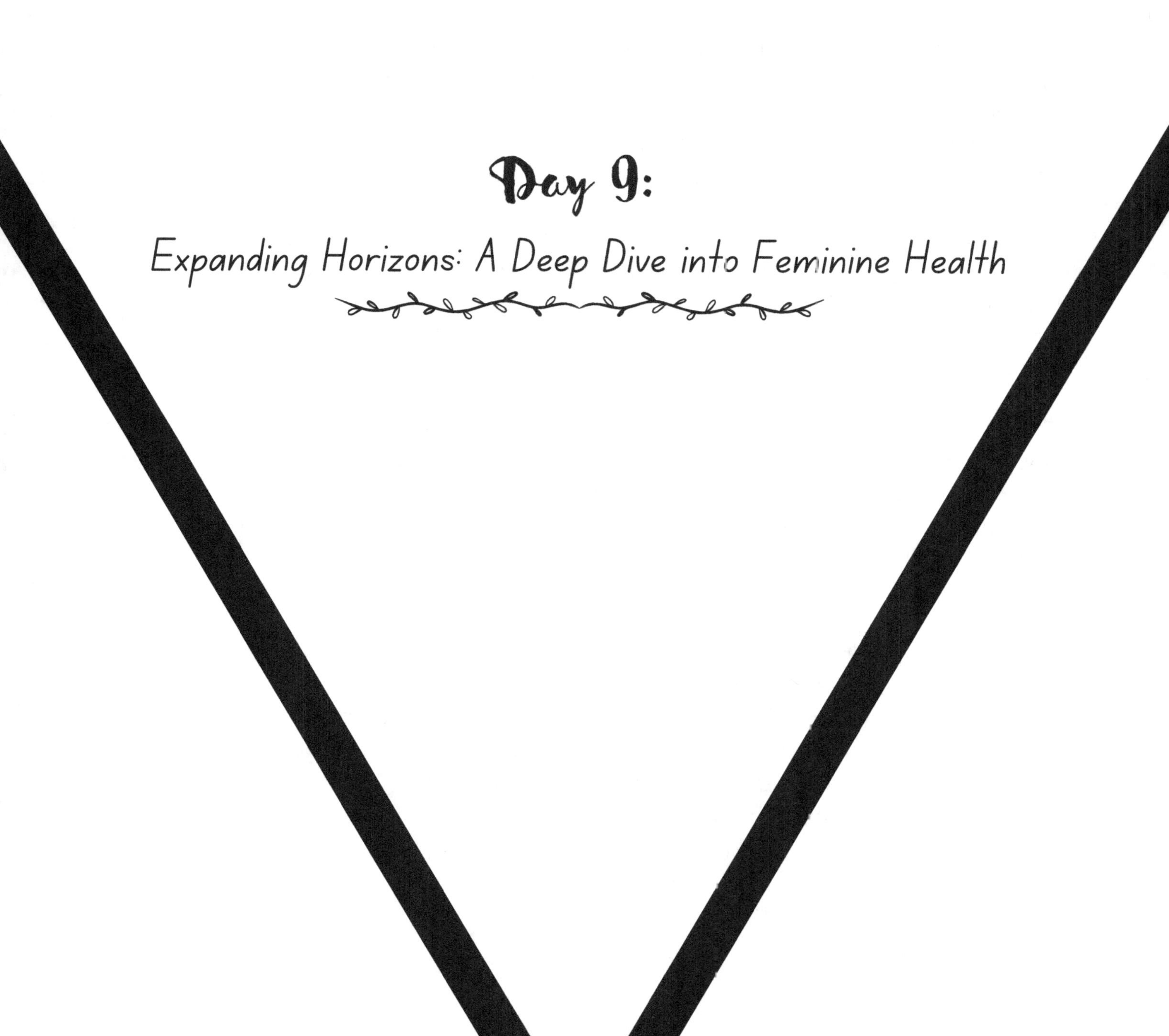

Day 9:

Expanding Horizons: A Deep Dive into Feminine Health

Day 9:

Expanding Horizons: A Deep Dive into Feminine Health

In this current era of easy access to information, it's crucial to continuously broaden our understanding of personal well-being. Feminine health, a topic that has been shrouded in mystery or misrepresented throughout history, is one such area that deserves our attention. Not only does comprehending our bodies lead to better physical health, but it also promotes mental well-being and confidence.

Exploring feminine health involves delving into a wide range of topics - from menstrual cycles and reproductive health to hormonal imbalances and the unique challenges that women face at different life stages. There is a complexity to the way our bodies function, a delicate balance of systems and a rhythmic dance of hormones, which have significant implications on our daily lives.

Taking the initiative to listen to a podcast or read an article on feminine health can be an eye-opening experience. Often, we are unaware of the intricacies within us until they are illuminated by experts in the field. With each new piece of information, there is a potential shift in perspective, a deeper respect for the body, and an understanding of its needs.

This knowledge is not only empowering for the individual but also for society as a whole. When women are educated about their bodies, they can advocate for better healthcare, make informed decisions, and dispel myths that have long perpetuated misunderstandings. Moreover, when women share their newfound knowledge with others, there is a ripple effect of empowerment, leading to a more informed and compassionate community.

In conclusion, feminine health is an ever-evolving field rich with insights that can transform our lives. By actively seeking knowledge through resources like podcasts or articles, we equip ourselves with the tools to navigate our health journey with confidence. As we embrace the affirmation "Knowledge empowers me," we are reminded of the strength that comes with understanding and the potential it has to reshape our relationship with our bodies.

<u>Self-Practice Activity for Day 9: "Journey Mapping"</u>

Objective: To encourage a deep, personal exploration of your own feminine health through various stages of life, recognizing patterns, and understanding shifts.

Instructions:

Materials Needed: A large sheet of paper or poster board, colored pens or pencils, stickers or images (optional).

Timeline Creation: Draw a horizontal line across the paper, representing your life's timeline from birth to your current age and beyond. Mark significant ages or periods, like the onset of menstruation, possible childbirth(s), or any other pivotal moments related to feminine health.

Life Events: Above the line, jot down significant life events or experiences that might have influenced or been influenced by your feminine health. It could be anything from your first period, a particular health challenge, or even an empowering conversation about women's health.

Physical and Emotional Notations: Below the line, note any physical changes, feelings, or emotions you experienced during these times. Were there hormonal shifts? How did they affect your mood or overall well-being?

Resources & Learnings: Allocate a section where you can list down resources (books, podcasts, articles) that you've found beneficial or wish to explore. As you go through them, jot down key takeaways.

Reflection: Once your map is complete, take a step back. What patterns do you observe? Are there certain periods where you wish you had more knowledge or support? Are there moments of empowerment and strength?

Engaging in this activity not only allows you to reflect on your own journey but also emphasizes the importance of continuous learning in the realm of feminine health. As you add to this map over time, it becomes a testament to your evolving understanding and the deep dive you're taking into the intricate world of feminine well-being.

Todays Affirmation:

"I honor and cherish the wisdom that comes with understanding my feminine health."

"Every step in my journey of feminine exploration strengthens my connection to myself."

"Knowledge empowers me, and with every discovery, I grow in confidence and grace."

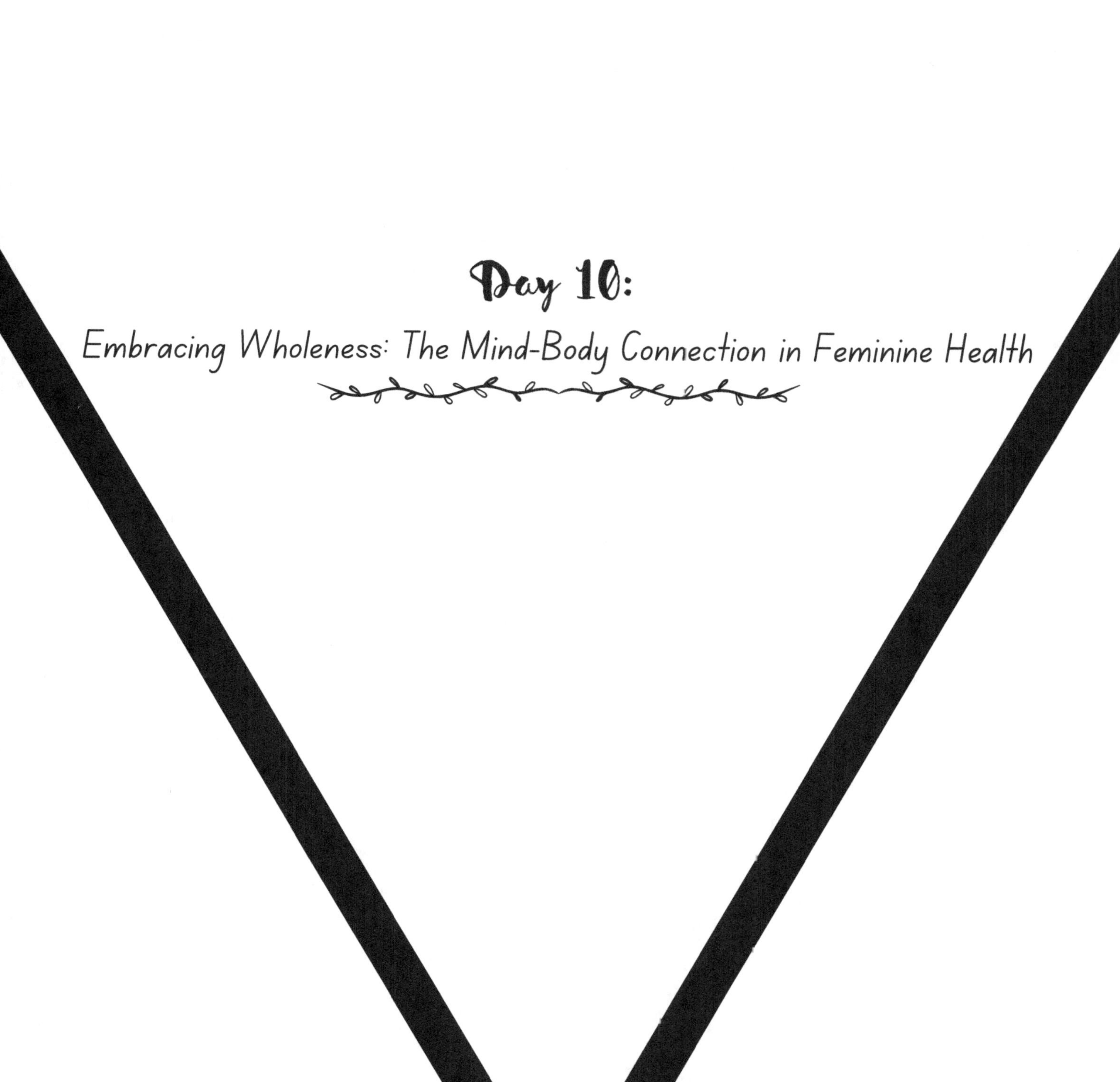

Day 10:

Embracing Wholeness: The Mind-Body Connection in Feminine Health

Day 10:

Embracing Wholeness: The Mind-Body Connection in Feminine Health

The symbiotic relationship between the mind and the body forms the crux of our overall well-being. Our mental state can influence our physical health, and vice versa. Especially in the realm of feminine health, understanding this interconnection is crucial. Today, we'll delve into the mind-body connection, learn how our thoughts and feelings influence our physical state, and explore practices that fortify both.

The Interwoven Threads of Mind and Body:

Emotions, thoughts, and stress levels can significantly impact our physical health. For instance, chronic stress may lead to hormonal imbalances, affecting menstrual cycles or inducing symptoms like fatigue. On the flip side, hormonal changes can influence our mood and cognitive functions.

Self-Care Tips:

- *Mindfulness Meditation:* Taking a few minutes daily to sit in silence, focusing on your breath or a specific thought, can reduce stress and bring clarity.

- *Physical Activity:* Engage in exercises that you enjoy, be it dancing, yoga, or jogging. Physical activity releases endorphins, often termed as 'feel-good hormones.'

- *Balanced Diet:* Consuming a nutrient-rich diet can bolster both mental and physical health. Omega-3 fatty acids, found in walnuts and flaxseeds, are known to support brain health.

Activities for the Day

- Body Scan Meditation: Lie down in a comfortable position. Starting from your toes, slowly bring awareness to each part of your body, noticing any sensations, tension, or warmth. This practice helps in grounding and connecting with your body.

- Journaling: Dedicate 15 minutes to write down your feelings, bodily sensations, and thoughts. Over time, you might notice patterns indicating how your mental state influences your physical well-being.

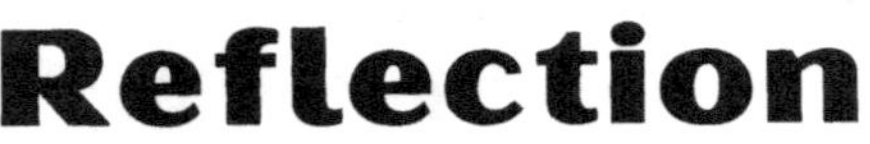

Reflection

1. Can you recall an instance where your mental state significantly impacted your physical well-being or vice versa?
2. What self-care practices resonate most with you in nurturing the mind-body connection?
3. How do you usually cope with stress, and how does it manifest in your body?

Todays Affirmation:

"Through mindfulness and attentive care, I honor both my body and mind as equally vital components of my vibrant health."

"With every breath and conscious thought, I fortify the bridge between my physical and mental well-being, creating harmony and balance."

"My mind and body are intricately connected, each supporting and nourishing the other on my journey to complete wellness."

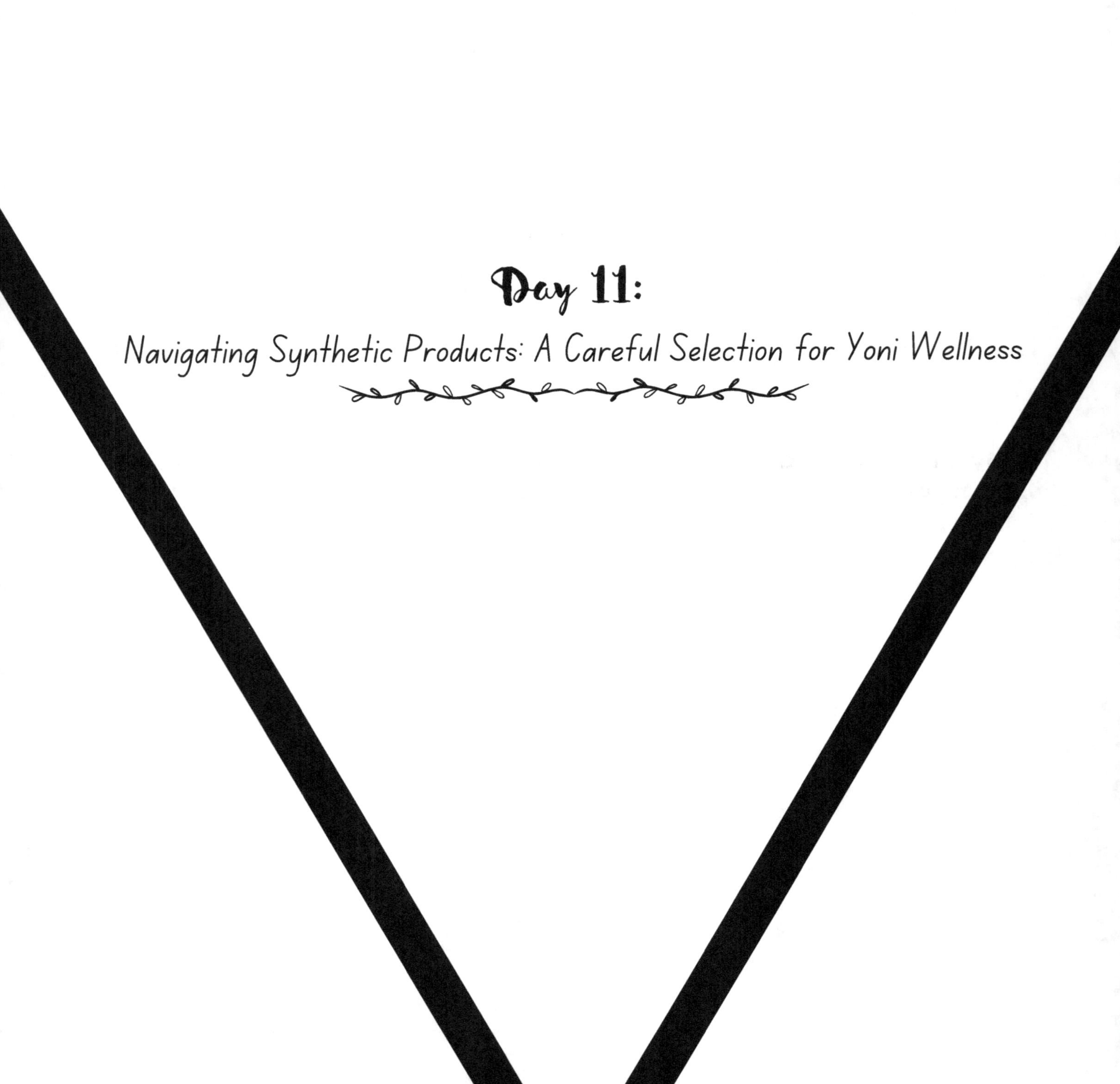

Day 11:

Navigating Synthetic Products: A Careful Selection for Yoni Wellness

Day 11:

Navigating Synthetic Products: A Careful Selection for Yoni Wellness

In a world abundant with products, making mindful selections for your yoni is crucial. Many items marketed for feminine hygiene contain synthetic ingredients that can be harsh or disruptive to the yoni's delicate balance. Day 11 guides you through understanding, selecting, and using products consciously, emphasizing safety and wellness.

Understanding the Risks:

- Many synthetic products, ranging from soaps and washes to menstrual products, often contain chemicals, fragrances, and dyes. These ingredients can:

- Cause irritation or allergic reactions.

- Disrupt the natural pH balance of the vagina.

- Lead to the development of yeast infections or bacterial vaginosis.

Tips for Mindful Selection:

- Read Labels: Pay attention to ingredients in any product you intend to use near your yoni. Avoid those with parabens, sulfates, and artificial fragrances.

- Opt for Hypoallergenic: Hypoallergenic products are designed to minimize allergic reactions, making them a safer choice for sensitive areas.

- Seek Professional Advice: If uncertain, consult with healthcare professionals to get recommendations based on your specific health profile and needs.

Activities for the Day:

Product Audit:

- *Purpose:* Review and evaluate the products you currently use.
- *How-To:* Gather all feminine hygiene products you have. Check their ingredient lists and discard those with harmful or irritating components.

Research & Education:

- *Purpose*: Equip yourself with knowledge.
- *How-To*: Spend some time researching reliable brands and products that are known for their safety and quality. Look for reviews and, if possible, scientific studies or expert opinions supporting their use.

Trial & Reflection:

- *Purpose:* Understand your body's reaction to different products.
- *How-To:* Introduce one new product at a time and observe how your body responds over several days. Document any discomfort, irritation, or satisfaction you experience.

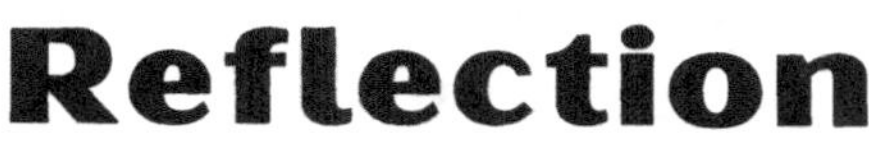

- Were there any products you were surprised to learn were not as safe as assumed?
- How does your body respond to the introduction of new, potentially safer products?
- Moving forward, how will you approach selecting products for your yoni's care?

Todays Affirmation:

"Informed and mindful, I choose products that align with the precious balance
and sanctity of my yoni's wellness."

"I am a conscious and informed guardian of my yoni's wellness, choosing products that
nurture rather than harm."

**"Each product I select is a testament to my commitment to nurturing
and protecting my feminine health with intention and respect."**

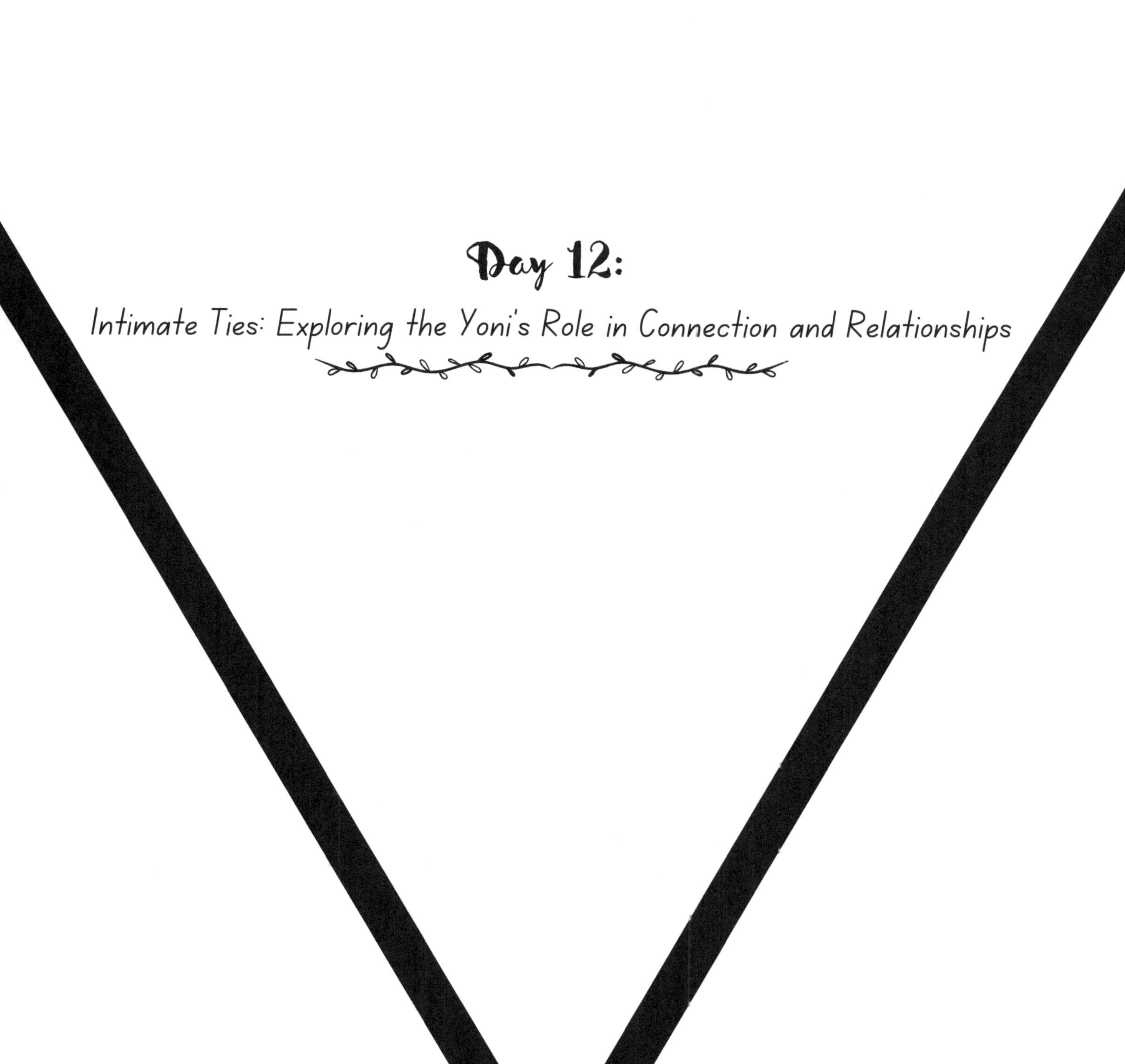

Day 12:

Intimate Ties: Exploring the Yoni's Role in Connection and Relationships

Day 12:

Intimate Ties: Exploring the Yoni's Role in Connection and Relationships

The yoni is not just a physical body part; it is closely connected with your emotional state, and it can impact and be impacted by your intimate connections and relationships. On Day 12, you are invited to delve into the various ways your yoni interacts with intimacy and how this affects your interpersonal relationships.

The Yoni & Intimacy: Deepening the Exploration

1. Physical Aspect:

- *Sensation and Pleasure*: The yoni is a complex network of nerve endings and sensitive tissues, providing the capability for intense pleasure and orgasm. This physical response not only enhances sexual enjoyment but also fosters a sense of closeness and connection with a partner.

- *Sexual Health and Function*: Conditions like dryness, infections, or other sexual health issues can affect intimate experiences. Understanding and addressing these issues is vital for enjoyable and pain-free intimacy.

2. Emotional Aspect:

- *Trust and Safety:* The yoni often responds to your emotional state. Feelings of safety and trust can lead to relaxation and receptiveness during intimacy, whereas fear or anxiety can result in tension or discomfort.

- *Emotional Memory:* The body, including the yoni, stores memories of past emotional experiences. Positive experiences can lead to anticipation and desire, while negative or traumatic experiences may result in fear, anxiety, or avoidance of intimacy.

3. **Energetic Aspect:**

- *Energetic Exchange:* Some spiritual and holistic practices believe in the exchange of energy during sexual intimacy. Your yoni's energy is believed to mingle with your partner's, potentially leading to a deeper connection or, conversely, to energy disturbances if the exchange is not consensual or respectful.

- *Chakra System:* In various traditions, the yoni is connected to the sacral chakra, the energy center related to sexuality, creativity, and emotions. Balancing and nurturing this chakra is thought to enhance your intimate and creative life.

4. **Psychological Aspect:**

- *Self-Image and Esteem*: How you perceive your yoni and sexuality plays a significant role in your intimate experiences. Positive self-image and confidence can enhance your intimate relationships, while insecurity or shame can hinder them.

- *Expectations and Beliefs:* Your beliefs about sexuality, intimacy, and what your yoni 'should' be like or 'should' experience can impact your sexual satisfaction and emotional well-being during intimate encounters.

Understanding for Healing and Growth:

It is important to develop a deeper understanding of the complex relationship between your yoni and intimacy. This understanding leads to healing, growth, and increased pleasure. Practicing self-reflection, seeking professional advice when necessary, and maintaining open communication with yourself and your partners are all crucial in nurturing this sacred aspect of your being. Whether you approach it from a medical, psychological, or spiritual perspective (or a combination of these), this understanding is essential for your overall well-being and the health of your intimate relationships.

Self-Reflection & Exploration: Insightful Journey into Intimacy

Self-reflection and exploration involve delving deeply into your inner world, perceptions, and experiences regarding intimacy. Understanding the interplay between your emotional and physical self provides insight into the dynamic relationship your yoni has with intimacy.

1. Yoni's Response to Intimacy:

- *Noticing Patterns*: Pay attention to how your yoni reacts in different intimate situations. Notice any patterns, like tightness or relaxation, pleasure or discomfort, in response to different stimuli or emotional states.

- *Physical Signs*: Be aware of physiological responses, such as arousal, lubrication, or sensitivity. These can be indicators of your comfort level and desire in intimate moments.

2. Emotional Connection:

- *Linking Emotions*: Explore the emotions that arise during intimate encounters. Joy, anxiety, vulnerability, and excitement might surface. Reflect on how these emotions correlate with your body's responses.

- *Past Experiences Impact*: Recognize that past emotional experiences, both positive and negative, influence your present perception and reaction to intimacy. Healing from negative experiences is crucial for enjoying and embracing future intimate moments.

3. Past Experiences and Learning:

Reflecting on Past Experiences: Take time to consider past intimate experiences, understanding their impact on how you currently view and engage in intimacy.

Learning and Unlearning: Reflection can bring awareness to beliefs and behaviors learned over time regarding intimacy and your yoni. Recognize which are helpful and which may need to be unlearned or redefined to foster a healthier intimate life.

4. Sensual Exploration Practice:

Engage in mindful, solo sensual exploration without the goal of orgasm but to understand what makes you feel good. This practice can help in creating a space for you to explore your desires and boundaries on your terms.

5. Intimacy Beliefs and Expectations:

Reflect on the beliefs and expectations you hold regarding intimacy and your yoni. How do these affect your experiences? Are these beliefs supportive of a fulfilling intimate life, or are they limiting?

The Importance of Reflection:
The act of self-reflection is empowering, allowing for self-discovery and the identification of areas that may need healing or growth. It fosters a deeper connection with yourself and improves your understanding of your needs and desires in intimacy.

Guided Reflection Activity:

Journaling Practice: Journaling can be a powerful tool for reflection. Write about your intimate experiences, thoughts, feelings, and reactions. Use prompts like:

- "How do I feel about my yoni during intimate moments?"
- "What emotions commonly arise during intimacy, and why?"
- "How have my past experiences shaped my approach to intimacy?"

Todays Affirmation:

"My yoni is a sacred space of connection and communication, actively participating in the dance of intimacy and relationships."

I embrace and honor the deep connection between my yoni and my heart, acknowledging the sacred dance they share in the realm of intimacy.

"I embrace and honor the deep connection between my yoni and my heart, acknowledging the sacred dance they share in the realm of intimacy."

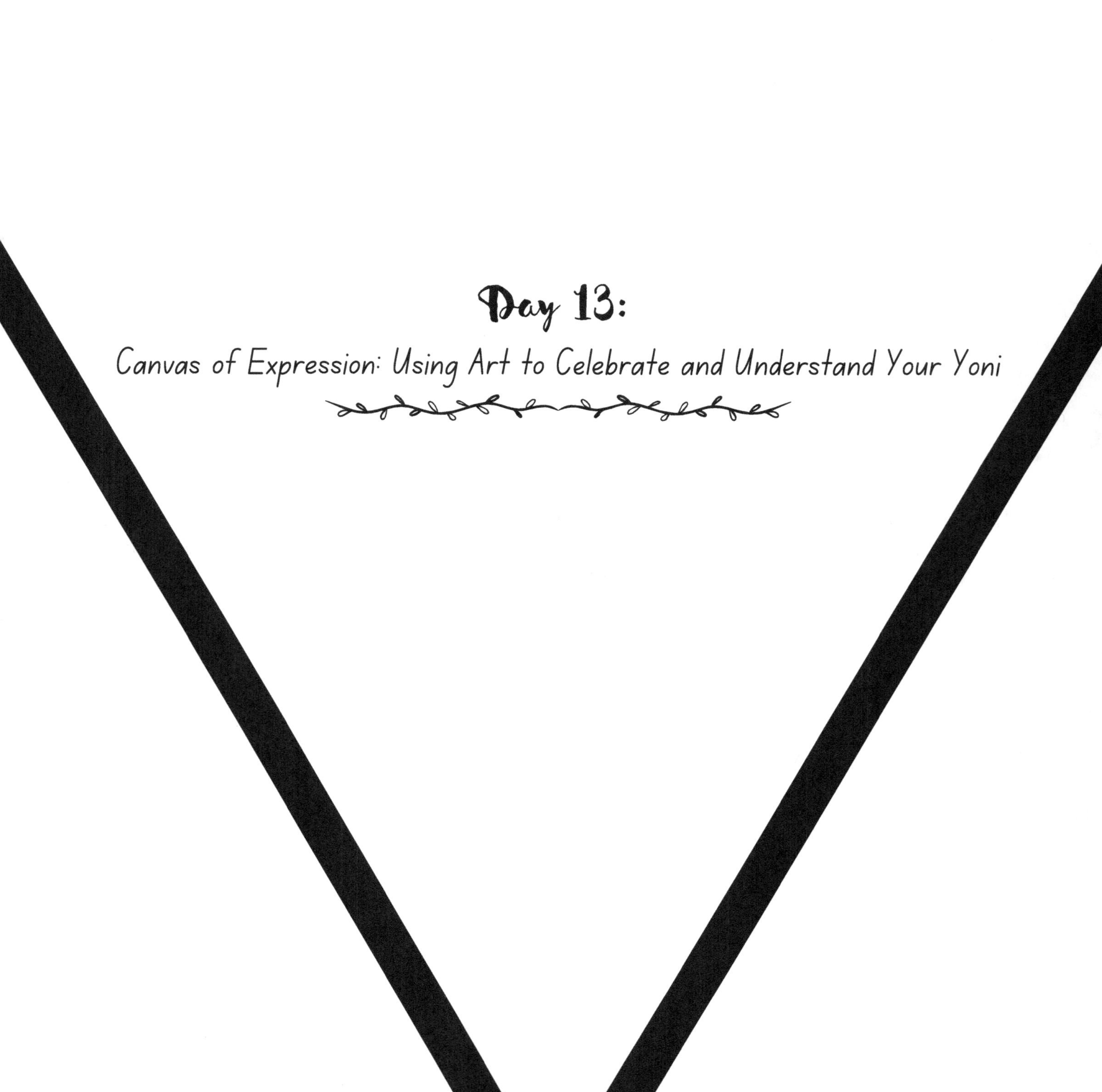

Day 13:

Canvas of Expression: Using Art to Celebrate and Understand Your Yoni

Day 13:

Canvas of Expression: Using Art to Celebrate and Understand Your Yoni

Art is a powerful medium that can be used for expression, healing, and celebration. It can offer deep insights into how you perceive, relate to, and feel about your yoni. On Day 13, we invite you to use different forms of art to explore and honor your relationship with your yoni. This will create a space for reflection, appreciation, and connection.

The Healing Power of Art and its Connection to the Yoni

Art is universally acknowledged for its transcendent healing capabilities, offering individuals a medium through which they can explore, understand, and celebrate their bodies, particularly the yoni. Through the lens of art, the yoni is not merely a physical organ but a symbol of divine femininity, strength, and sensuality.

Firstly, art serves as an expressive outlet facilitating emotional release. Engaging with art allows women to communicate their deepest feelings, fears, joys, and experiences related to their yonis without needing to articulate them verbally. In a society where discussions around feminine anatomy can sometimes be stifled, art provides a voice, enabling women to share their stories of pleasure, pain, childbirth, menstrual experiences, and more. This process of externalizing one's intimate emotions fosters catharsis and emotional unburdening, promoting mental health.

Moreover, Art has the power to enhance self-understanding and connection with one's yoni through visualization and representation. Every stroke, color choice, and material selected to depict the yoni in art reflects the creator's perception, relationship, and emotions towards it. By engaging in this introspective process, women can reflect on their self-image, sexuality, and identity. Celebrating the yoni through visual art helps to break down societal stigmas and fosters a sense of pride and respect for the feminine form.

Furthermore, art plays a pivotal role in healing. For those carrying traumas or negative experiences related to their yonis, engaging with art can be therapeutic. Through creation, they can navigate through these emotions, finding a path towards healing and acceptance. Art not only assists in reconciling with past pains but also in envisaging a future of empowerment and positive sexuality.

Finally, the interaction with art engenders community building. Viewing and reflecting upon yoni art created by others fosters a sense of solidarity and shared experience among women. It aids in realizing that each woman's experience is unique yet intertwined in the collective feminine narrative.

In conclusion, the marriage between art and the yoni is a harmonious alliance that fosters expression, healing, and celebration of femininity. Through the canvas, brush, or clay, women find a conduit for healing and a platform for celebration, weaving a tapestry that honors the sacredness and strength of the yoni. The healing power of art, in this context, is indeed a beacon of transformation and empowerment for every woman.

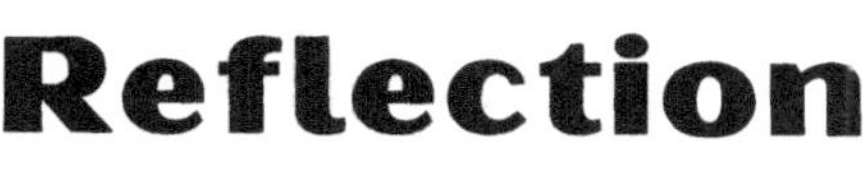

Reflection

- What emotions emerged during the art creation process?
- How does the final artwork represent your connection with your yoni?
- Did the artistic process provide any new insights or perspectives regarding your yoni and femininity?

Todays Affirmation:

"My yoni is a masterpiece of beauty, strength, and mystery, worthy of celebration and deep appreciation through the canvas of expression."

"Through art, I connect deeply with my yoni, celebrating its essence and honoring its profound narratives."

"Each brushstroke and hue is a testament to the power, beauty, and resilience of my feminine spirit."

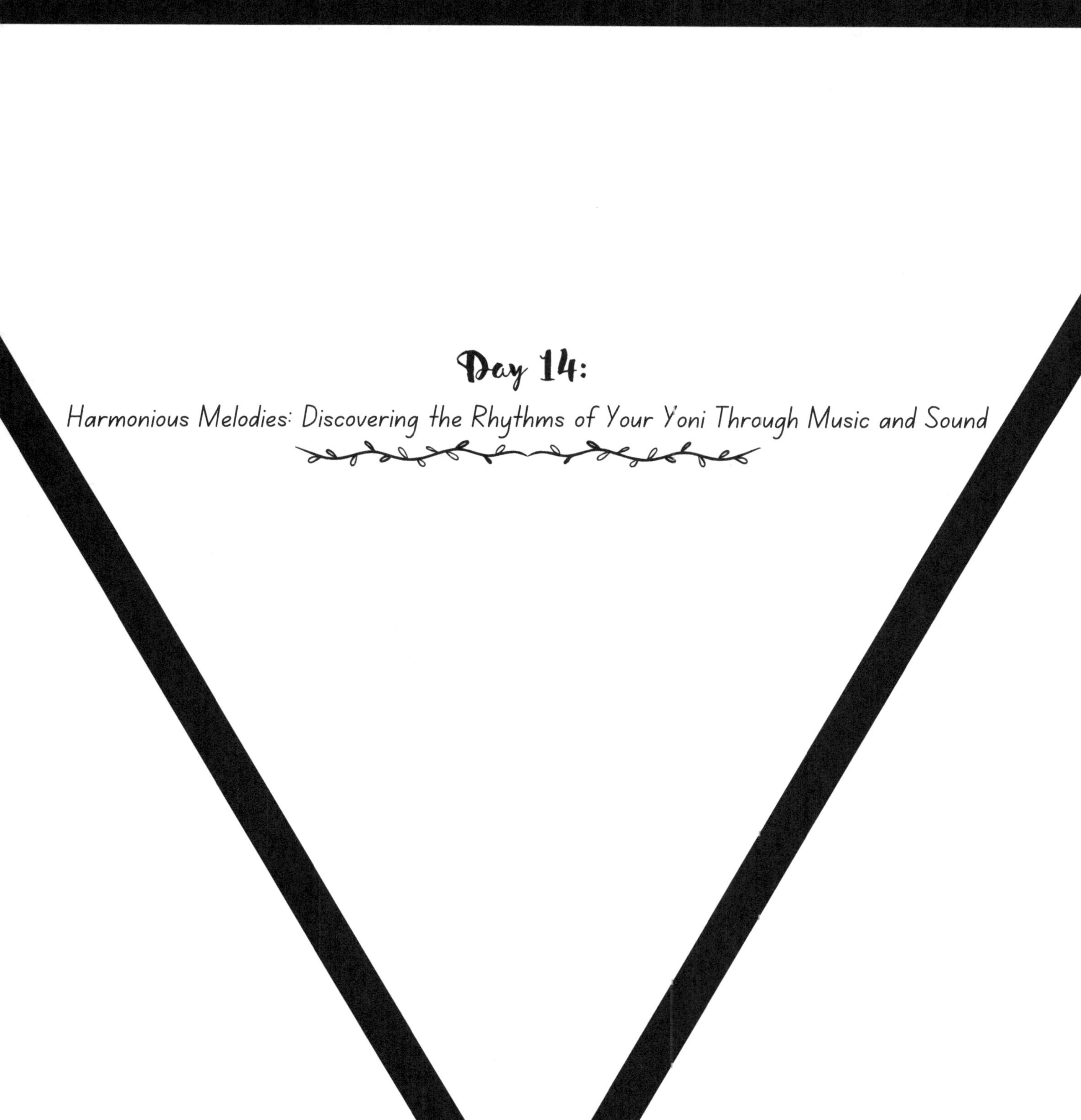

Day 14:

Harmonious Melodies: Discovering the Rhythms of Your Yoni Through Music and Sound

Day 14:

Harmonious Melodies: Discovering the Rhythms of Your Yoni Through Music and Sound

Music and sound have been integral parts of healing and celebration in various cultures. Their rhythm, melody, and harmony can reflect and influence our emotions and bodily responses. Day 14 is dedicated to exploring how music and sound resonate with the energies and rhythms of your yoni, offering an auditory canvas to express, celebrate, and understand your feminine essence.

The Symphony of Music & the Yoni:

- *Vibrational Energy:* Music carries vibrational energies that can align with or influence the energies of your body, including the yoni. Engaging with music can offer relaxation, arousal, or emotional release.

- *Expression and Emotion:* Different musical genres and pieces can evoke or mirror the vast range of emotions and experiences associated with the yoni, providing an auditory language for expression.

- *Healing and Soothing:* Sound healing and music therapy have been shown to reduce stress and promote healing, offering a supportive tool for overall yoni wellness.

My Yoni Bath Soak

♡ Take some time tonight to pamper your yoni with a soothing bath and some relaxing tunes. Create a playlist to enhance her experience.

♡ Make a Playlist For Tonight's Bath:

____

____

____

____

♡ Bath Soak Recipe For My Yoni

Ingredients:

1 cup Epsom salt
1/2 cup baking soda
5 drops of lavender essential oil
5 drops of chamomile essential oil
1/4 cup dried rose petals (optional)

Directions:

1. Fill your bathtub with warm water.
2. As the tub fills, sprinkle in the Epsom salt and baking soda, allowing them to dissolve.
3. Once dissolved, add the essential oils and stir the water gently to distribute them evenly.
4. If desired, sprinkle in dried rose petals for an added touch of luxury and calm.
5. Soak for 20-30 minutes, breathing deeply and allowing the soothing properties of the ingredients to permeate your skin and relax the yoni.

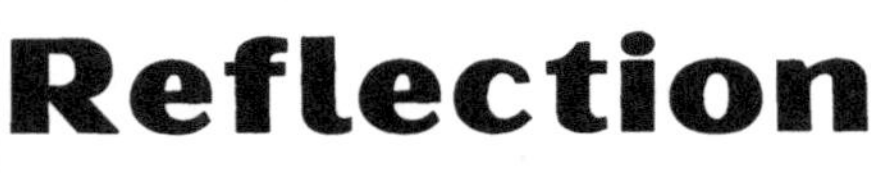

Reflection

1. How does music influence your perception or feeling towards your yoni?
2. Did any particular genre or piece of music evoke strong reactions or alignment with your yoni?
3. How can incorporating music and sound into your routine support your yoni wellness?

Todays Affirmation:

"The symphony of life plays harmoniously with my feminine essence,
creating a melody of love, empowerment, and joy in my soul."

"With every note and rhythm, I attune to the sacred dance within, celebrating the music
that emanates from my yoni's divine energy."

**"In the dance of melodies and harmonies, I find a sonic
reflection of my yoni's beauty, strength, and depth,
moving gracefully to the rhythm of life."**

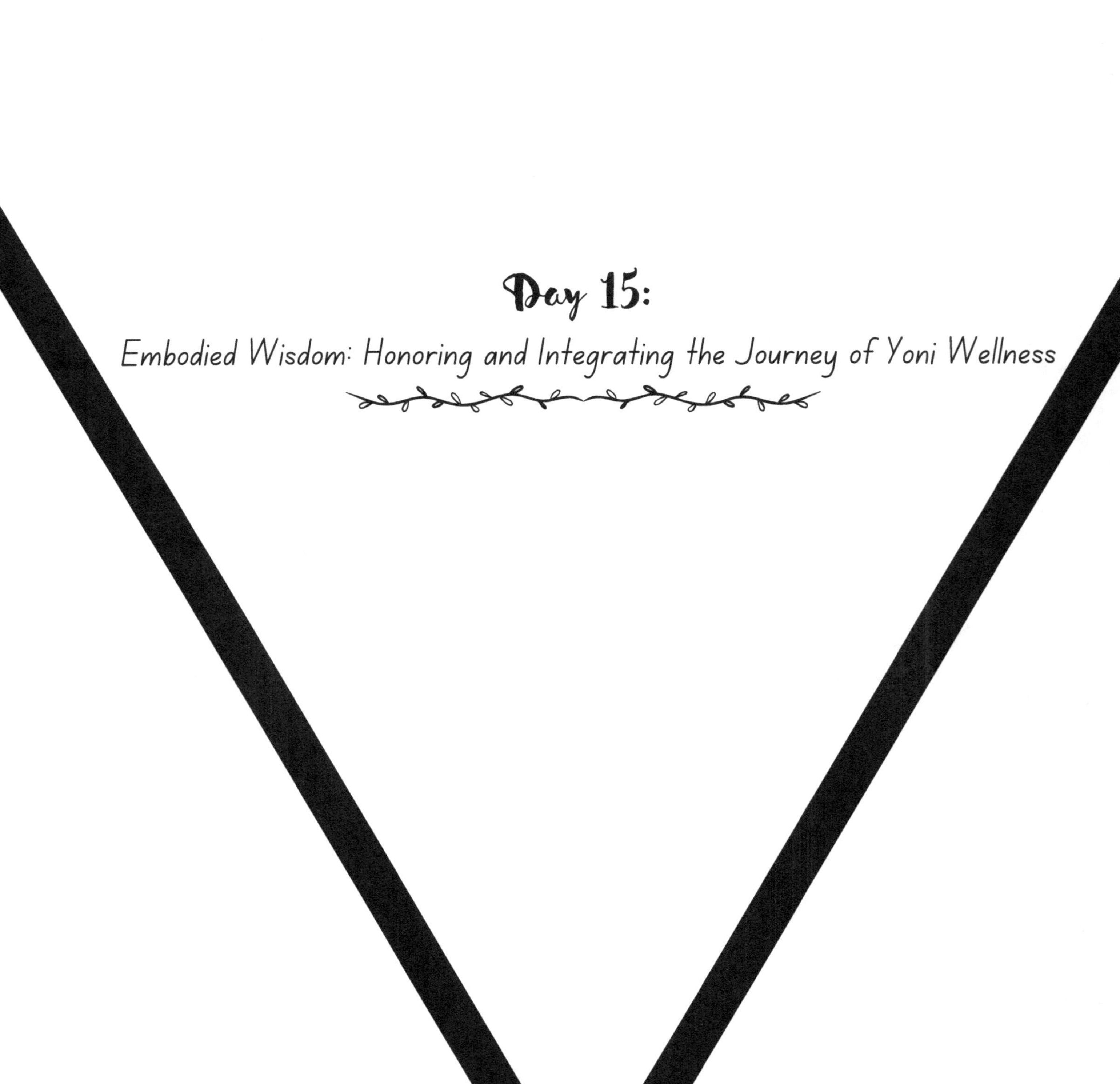

Day 15:

Embodied Wisdom: Honoring and Integrating the Journey of Yoni Wellness

Day 15:

Embodied Wisdom: Honoring and Integrating the Journey of Yoni Wellness

As we arrive at the closing chapter of this journey, Day 15 is dedicated to reflecting on, honoring, and integrating the wisdom and insights you've gathered throughout the preceding days. It's a day for celebration, acknowledgment, and forward-looking inspiration towards continued Yoni wellness.

Self Tips:

1. *Consistent Practice:*

- The journey doesn't end here; maintaining Yoni wellness requires consistent attention and practice. Continue with the activities and reflections that resonated most with you.

2. *Listen Intently:*

- Your yoni speaks; it's crucial to listen. Pay attention to its signals, acknowledging when it needs care, rest, healing, or celebration.

3. *Seek Professional Advice:*

- For any health concerns or deeper emotional healing related to Yoni wellness, don't hesitate to consult healthcare professionals or counselors.

Resources:

1. *Books:*

- Look for books on women's health, sexuality, and spirituality that provide deeper insights into the mysteries and mechanics of the yoni.

2. *Online Platforms:*

- Engage with reputable websites, forums, and social media groups dedicated to feminine health and wellness for community support and additional resources.

3. *Workshops & Retreats:*

- Consider attending workshops, retreats, or seminars focused on feminine energy, sexuality, and holistic wellness.

Meditation Tips:

1. *Daily Mindfulness:*

- Incorporate mindfulness or meditation practices into your daily routine, focusing on connecting with and honoring your yoni.

2. *Visualization:*

- Engage in meditations that involve visualizing healing, loving energy enveloping your yoni, and promoting wellness and balance.

3. *Guided Meditations:*

- Explore guided meditations and sound healings dedicated to Yoni wellness and feminine energy available online or in meditation apps.

<u>Self Activity: Reflection and Vision Board Creation</u>

Objective:

Reflect on the journey and envision the future of your Yoni wellness.

Instructions:

1. *Reflect:*

- Consider the significant insights, healing moments, and celebrations experienced during the past 14 days.

2. *Envision:*

- Visualize your path forward in maintaining and deepening the connection with your yoni.

3. *Create a Vision Board:*

- Use images, words, or symbols to represent your reflections and visions regarding your Yoni wellness on a board. Place it where you can see it regularly as a reminder and inspiration.

As the sun sets on Day 15, it marks not an end, but a beautiful beginning, a continual dance of discovery, reverence, and care for your yoni. The journey traversed has hopefully sown seeds of understanding, love, and appreciation for your unique feminine essence. Embark forward armed with knowledge, imbued with love, and radiant with the sacred energy of your yoni. The canvas of life awaits your vibrant colors of wisdom, strength, and joy derived from the wellspring of yoni wellness. Celebrate each day as a symphony of harmonious melodies, a masterpiece painted with the hues of your embodied wisdom, and a sacred narrative written in the ink of your experiences. The journey continues, and so does the dance – beautifully, powerfully, and sacredly.

"Embarking on the endless journey of self-discovery and yoni wellness, I carry with me a tapestry of wisdom, strength, and love, weaving a narrative that is uniquely mine, infinitely powerful, and deeply sacred."

As you gently close the pages of this book, may you continue to unfold the sacred pages of your own story, nurturing, celebrating, and honoring the divine yoni that resides within you, guiding you through the dance of life with grace, wisdom, and boundless love."

My Notes:

My Notes:

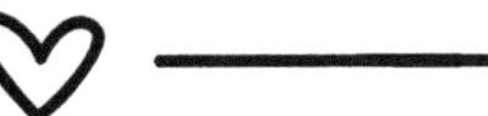

My Notes:

My Notes:

My Notes:

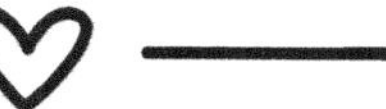

My Notes:

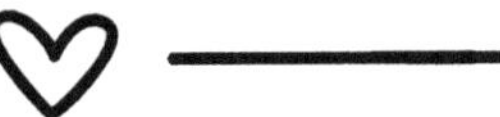

My Notes:

My Notes: